ULTIMATE GUIDE
TO
JUICE CLEANSES

DETOX, HEALTH BENEFITS, AND RECIPES

By

Dr. Graceful Aging

Copyright

Table Of Contents

CHAPTER 1: INTRODUCTION TO JUICE CLEANSES

What is a Juice Cleanse?

History and Popularity of Juice Cleanses

Common Myths and Misconceptions

CHAPTER 2: Health Benefits of Juice Cleanses

Detoxification and Cleansing

Boosting Immunity

Improving Digestion

Weight Loss and Metabolism Enhancement

Enhancing Skin Health

Conclusion

CHAPTER 3: TYPES OF JUICE CLEANSES

One-Day Cleanse

Three-Day Cleanse

Five-Day Cleanse

Customizable Cleanses

Conclusion**

CHAPTER 4: PREPARING FOR A JUICE CLEANSE

Setting Realistic Goals

Shopping List and Ingredients

Necessary Equipment (Juicers, Blenders)

Pre-Cleanse Diet Tips

CHAPTER 5: JUICE CLEANSE RECIPES

Green Detox Juice

Citrus Immunity Booster

Berry Antioxidant Blend

Refreshing Hydration Mix

Protein-Packed Vegetable Juice

Conclusion

CHAPTER 6: DURING THE CLEANSE

Daily Schedule and Routine

Managing Hunger and Cravings

Staying Hydrated

Monitoring Your Body's Responses

Conclusion

CHAPTER 7: POST-CLEANSE: TRANSITIONING BACK TO SOLID FOODS

Gradual Reintroduction of Solid Foods

Maintaining Benefits of the Cleanse

Long-Term Healthy Eating Habits

Example Post-Cleanse Meal Plan

CHAPTER 8: POTENTIAL RISKS AND CONSIDERATIONS

Who Should Avoid Juice Cleanses

Common Side Effects and How to Mitigate Them

Consulting with Healthcare Professionals

Conclusion

CHAPTER 9: SUCCESS STORIES AND TESTIMONIALS

Real-Life Experiences

Tips from Juice Cleanse Veterans

Conclusion

CHAPTER 10: FAQs ABOUT JUICE CLEANSES

RESOURCES AND FURTHER READING

Recommended Books and Articles
Online Communities and Support Groups
Additional Recipes and Meal Plans
Conclusion

CHAPTER 1: INTRODUCTION TO JUICE CLEANSES

What is a Juice Cleanse?

A juice cleanse is a type of detox diet that involves consuming only fruit and vegetable juices for a specific period, typically ranging from one to five days. The primary goal of a juice cleanse is to detoxify the body, improve digestion, and promote overall health by providing a concentrated source of nutrients while giving the digestive system a break from solid foods.

During a juice cleanse, individuals consume a variety of freshly prepared juices, which may include a mix of fruits, vegetables, herbs, and spices. These juices are designed to be nutrientdense, rich in vitamins, minerals, antioxidants, and phytonutrients. The idea is that by consuming these nutrientpacked juices, the body can eliminate toxins, reduce inflammation, and improve energy levels and mental clarity.

Juice cleanses are typically divided into three phases: preparation, the cleanse itself, and postcleanse. The preparation phase involves gradually eliminating certain foods from the diet, such as caffeine, alcohol, refined sugars, and processed foods, to ease the transition into the cleanse. During the cleanse, individuals consume only the prescribed juices, herbal teas, and water. The postcleanse phase involves reintroducing solid foods gradually, starting with easily digestible foods like fruits, vegetables, and whole grains.

Proponents of juice cleanses claim that they offer numerous health benefits, including improved digestion, weight loss, enhanced immune function, increased energy levels, clearer skin, and mental clarity. However, it is essential to approach juice cleanses with caution and be aware of the potential risks and limitations, especially for those with certain medical conditions or nutritional needs.

History and Popularity of Juice Cleanses

The concept of juice cleansing is not new and can be traced back to ancient civilizations that practiced fasting and detoxification rituals. In ancient Greece, fasting was often used as a means of purifying the body and mind. Similarly, Ayurvedic and Traditional Chinese Medicine systems have long promoted the use of herbal and plantbased remedies to support detoxification and overall health.

The modern juice cleanse movement gained traction in the early 20th century, with the rise of naturopathy and the promotion of raw food diets. Pioneers like Dr. Norman Walker, who is credited with popularizing juicing, advocated for the consumption of fresh vegetable and fruit juices as a means of improving health and longevity. His book, "Fresh Vegetable and Fruit Juices," published in 1936, remains a foundational text for those interested in the benefits of juicing.

The 1990s and early 2000s saw a resurgence in the popularity of juice cleanses, driven in part by the growing interest in holistic health and wellness. The rise of the internet and social media played a significant role in spreading information and testimonials about the benefits of juice cleanses. Celebrities and influencers began to endorse juice cleanses as a way to achieve quick weight loss, glowing skin, and increased energy, further fueling their popularity.

Juice bars and cleanse programs started to emerge, offering prepackaged juice cleanses that made it easier for individuals to embark on a cleanse without having to prepare the juices themselves. Companies like BluePrint Cleanse, Pressed Juicery, and Suja Juice became household names, providing a wide range of juice cleanse options to cater to different needs and preferences.

Despite the popularity of juice cleanses, they have also faced criticism and skepticism from the medical and scientific communities. Critics argue that the body already has natural detoxification systems in place, such as the liver and kidneys, and that there is limited scientific evidence to support the claimed benefits of juice cleanses. Additionally, some nutritionists caution that juice cleanses can be low in protein and fiber, leading to potential nutrient deficiencies if done for extended periods.

Common Myths and Misconceptions

The rise of juice cleanses has also led to the proliferation of myths and misconceptions surrounding their benefits and potential drawbacks. Understanding these myths is crucial for making informed decisions about whether a juice cleanse is right for you.

Myth 1: Juice Cleanses Detoxify Your Body

One of the most pervasive myths about juice cleanses is that they detoxify the body by flushing out toxins. While it's true that consuming nutrientrich juices can support the body's natural detoxification processes, the notion that juice cleanses alone can remove toxins is oversimplified. The liver, kidneys, and other organs are already efficient at detoxifying the body, and there is limited scientific evidence to suggest that juice cleanses significantly enhance this process.

Myth 2: Juice Cleanses Lead to Permanent Weight Loss

Another common misconception is that juice cleanses are a quick fix for weight loss. While it's possible to lose weight during a juice cleanse due to the lowcalorie intake, this weight loss is often temporary and primarily due to water loss and reduced muscle mass. Once solid foods are reintroduced, the weight is likely to return. Sustainable weight loss requires longterm lifestyle changes, including a balanced diet and regular exercise.

Myth 3: Juice Cleanses Provide All the Nutrients You Need

Juice cleanses can be nutrientdense, but they are often low in essential macronutrients like protein and healthy fats. While juices can provide vitamins, minerals, and antioxidants, they typically lack the fiber found in whole fruits and vegetables. Fiber is crucial for digestive health and helps regulate blood sugar levels. Additionally, the absence of protein in most juice cleanses can lead to muscle loss and decreased energy levels. For a balanced diet, it's important to consume a variety of whole foods that provide all necessary nutrients.

Myth 4: Juice Cleanses Improve Digestive Health

Some proponents claim that juice cleanses give the digestive system a break and improve gut health. However, the lack of fiber in juices can actually have the opposite effect. Fiber is essential for maintaining healthy bowel movements and supporting gut microbiota. Extended juice cleanses can lead to digestive issues such as constipation or diarrhea. For optimal digestive health, a diet rich in fiber from whole fruits, vegetables, and whole grains is recommended.

Myth 5: Juice Cleanses Are Suitable for Everyone

While juice cleanses can be beneficial for some individuals, they are not suitable for everyone. People with certain medical conditions, such as diabetes, kidney disease, or eating disorders, should avoid juice cleanses due to potential health risks. Pregnant or breastfeeding women, children, and individuals with compromised immune systems should also refrain from juice cleanses. It's essential to consult with a healthcare professional before starting a juice cleanse, especially if you have any underlying health conditions.

Myth 6: All Juices Are Equally Beneficial

Not all juices are created equal. The nutritional content of juices can vary significantly depending on the ingredients used and the method of preparation. Coldpressed juices, which are made using hydraulic presses, retain more nutrients and enzymes compared to juices made with centrifugal juicers. Additionally, juices high in fruits can be high in natural sugars, leading to spikes in blood sugar levels. Balancing fruit juices with vegetable juices can help maintain stable blood sugar levels and provide a wider range of nutrients.

Myth 7: Juice Cleanses Are the Best Way to Reset Your Body

While juice cleanses can provide a mental and physical reset for some individuals, they are not the only or necessarily the best way to achieve this. Other methods, such as mindful eating, regular physical activity, adequate sleep, and stress management, can also contribute to a sense of rejuvenation and wellbeing. A holistic approach to health and wellness that includes a balanced diet and lifestyle changes is often more sustainable and effective in the long term.

In conclusion, juice cleanses have a rich history and have gained popularity for their potential health benefits. However, it's important to approach them with a critical mindset and be aware of the common myths and misconceptions. Juice cleanses can offer a temporary boost in nutrients and a mental reset, but they should not be relied upon as a quick fix for detoxification or weight loss. Consulting with a healthcare professional and incorporating juice cleanses as part of a balanced and holistic approach to health is essential for achieving optimal results.

CHAPTER 2: Health Benefits of Juice Cleanses

Detoxification and Cleansing

Detoxification and cleansing are among the most touted benefits of juice cleanses. The idea is that by consuming only nutrientdense juices, the body can eliminate toxins more efficiently. This process is believed to reset and rejuvenate the body's natural detoxification systems.

How Detoxification Works

The body has several builtin mechanisms to detoxify itself, primarily through the liver, kidneys, lungs, skin, and gastrointestinal tract. These organs work together to process and eliminate harmful substances, including environmental pollutants, metabolic waste products, and toxins from food and beverages.

Liver: The liver is the body's primary detoxification organ. It filters the blood, metabolizes toxins, and converts them into less harmful substances that can be excreted.

Kidneys: The kidneys filter waste products and excess substances from the blood, which are then excreted in the urine.

Lungs: The lungs expel carbon dioxide and other volatile compounds during respiration.

Skin: The skin eliminates toxins through sweat.

Gastrointestinal Tract: The digestive system processes food, absorbs nutrients, and eliminates waste products through bowel movements.

Role of Juice Cleanses in Detoxification

Proponents of juice cleanses argue that by consuming only liquids, the digestive system gets a break from processing solid foods, allowing the body to focus more on detoxification. Additionally, the high intake of vitamins, minerals, and antioxidants from juices is believed to support the body's natural detox processes. Ingredients commonly used in juice cleanses, such as leafy greens, citrus fruits, and herbs, are rich in compounds that may enhance liver function and promote detoxification.

Leafy Greens: Vegetables like kale, spinach, and parsley are high in chlorophyll, which is thought to help remove toxins and support liver health.

Citrus Fruits: Lemons, limes, and oranges are rich in vitamin C, an antioxidant that aids in the detoxification process.

Herbs: Ingredients like ginger and turmeric have antiinflammatory and antioxidant properties that may support detoxification.

Scientific Evidence

While many people report feeling refreshed and rejuvenated after a juice cleanse, scientific evidence supporting the detoxification claims is limited. Some studies suggest that certain ingredients in juices can support liver health and antioxidant status, but more research is needed to confirm these effects. It's essential to recognize that the body is already equipped with efficient detoxification systems and that a balanced diet and healthy lifestyle are crucial for maintaining these processes.

Boosting Immunity

A strong immune system is vital for protecting the body against infections, diseases, and other health issues. Juice cleanses are often promoted as a way to boost immunity by providing a concentrated source of vitamins, minerals, and antioxidants that support immune function.

Key Nutrients for Immune Health

Vitamin C: An essential nutrient found in citrus fruits, berries, and leafy greens, vitamin C is known for its immuneboosting properties. It helps stimulate the production of white blood cells, which are crucial for fighting infections.

Vitamin A: Found in carrots, sweet potatoes, and leafy greens, vitamin A supports the immune system by maintaining the health of the skin and mucous membranes, which act as barriers to pathogens.

Vitamin E: This antioxidant, present in nuts, seeds, and green leafy vegetables, helps protect cells from oxidative stress and supports immune function.

Zinc: An essential mineral found in small amounts in juices containing spinach, pumpkin seeds, and other vegetables, zinc is important for immune cell development and function.

Antioxidants: Compounds found in fruits and vegetables, such as flavonoids and polyphenols, help reduce inflammation and oxidative stress, which can weaken the immune system.

Role of Juice Cleanses in Boosting Immunity

Juice cleanses provide a high intake of these immuneboosting nutrients in an easily digestible form. By consuming a variety of fruits and vegetables, individuals can enhance their intake of essential vitamins and minerals that support immune function. The antioxidants present in juices help combat free radicals and reduce inflammation, further supporting overall health and immunity.

Scientific Evidence

While there is evidence that a diet rich in fruits and vegetables can support immune health, specific research on juice cleanses and immunity is limited. Some studies have shown that increasing the intake of certain vitamins and antioxidants can enhance immune function, but more research is needed to determine the direct effects of juice cleanses on the immune system. It's important to note that maintaining a balanced diet and a healthy lifestyle is crucial for longterm immune health.

Improving Digestion

Proper digestion is essential for overall health and wellbeing. Juice cleanses are often promoted as a way to improve digestion by giving the digestive system a break from processing solid foods and providing easily absorbable nutrients.

Benefits of Juice Cleanses for Digestion

Resting the Digestive System: By consuming only liquids, the digestive system can take a break from breaking down complex foods, potentially reducing digestive stress and allowing for more efficient nutrient absorption.

Hydration: Juices are high in water content, which helps maintain hydration levels and supports digestive health. Proper hydration is essential for the production of digestive juices and the smooth movement of food through the digestive tract.

Enzymes: Freshly prepared juices contain natural enzymes that aid in digestion. These enzymes can help break down food and improve nutrient absorption.

Detoxification: Certain ingredients in juices, such as ginger and lemon, have been shown to support liver function and promote detoxification, which can indirectly benefit digestion.

Potential Drawbacks

Lack of Fiber: One of the primary drawbacks of juice cleanses is the lack of dietary fiber, which is essential for healthy digestion. Fiber helps regulate bowel movements, supports gut health, and prevents constipation. Most juices lack the fiber found in whole fruits and vegetables, which can lead to digestive issues if the cleanse is prolonged.

Blood Sugar Spikes: Juices high in fruit content can lead to rapid spikes in blood sugar levels, which can negatively impact digestive health and overall wellbeing. Balancing fruit juices with vegetable juices can help mitigate this effect.

Scientific Evidence

While juice cleanses may provide a temporary break for the digestive system and offer easily absorbable nutrients, the longterm benefits for digestion are unclear. A balanced diet rich in whole foods, including fruits, vegetables, whole grains, and fiber, is essential for maintaining optimal digestive health. Incorporating juices as part of a balanced diet, rather than relying solely on juice cleanses, is likely more beneficial for digestion.

Weight Loss and Metabolism Enhancement

Weight loss is one of the most commonly cited reasons for embarking on a juice cleanse. The lowcalorie nature of juice cleanses can lead to rapid weight loss, but it's important to understand the nuances and potential implications of this approach.

ShortTerm Weight Loss

Caloric Deficit: Juice cleanses typically involve consuming fewer calories than usual, leading to a caloric deficit that results in weight loss. This initial weight loss is often due to the reduction in water retention and glycogen stores, rather than fat loss.

Reduced Bloating: The high water content and lack of solid foods can reduce bloating and water retention, leading to a slimmer appearance and temporary weight loss.

LongTerm Weight Loss and Metabolism

Sustainability: While juice cleanses can lead to shortterm weight loss, maintaining this weight loss can be challenging once solid foods are reintroduced. Sustainable weight loss requires longterm dietary and lifestyle changes, including a balanced diet and regular exercise.

Muscle Loss: The lack of protein in most juice cleanses can lead to muscle loss, which can negatively impact metabolism. Muscle mass is essential for maintaining a healthy metabolic rate, and losing muscle can slow down metabolism, making it harder to maintain weight loss.

Metabolic Adaptation: Prolonged calorie restriction can lead to metabolic adaptation, where the body adjusts to a lower calorie intake by reducing its metabolic rate. This adaptation can make it more challenging to lose weight and maintain weight loss over time.

Scientific Evidence

Research on the longterm effects of juice cleanses on weight loss and metabolism is limited. While juice cleanses can provide a shortterm weight loss solution, they are not a sustainable approach for longterm weight management. A balanced diet that includes adequate protein, healthy fats, and fiber, combined with regular physical activity, is essential for achieving and maintaining a healthy weight and metabolism.

Enhancing Skin Health

Clear, glowing skin is often considered a sign of good health and is another reason why many people turn to juice cleanses. The high nutrient content and hydration provided by juices are believed to support skin health and improve its appearance.

Nutrients for Skin Health

Vitamin C: An antioxidant that supports collagen production, vitamin C helps maintain skin elasticity and reduce the appearance of wrinkles. Citrus fruits, berries, and leafy greens are excellent sources of vitamin C.

Vitamin A: This vitamin promotes skin cell turnover and repair, helping to maintain smooth and healthy skin. Carrots, sweet potatoes, and leafy greens are rich in vitamin A.

Vitamin E: An antioxidant that protects the skin from oxidative damage, vitamin E is found in nuts, seeds, and green leafy vegetables.

BetaCarotene: A precursor to vitamin A, betacarotene helps protect the skin from UV damage and supports overall skin health. Carrots, sweet potatoes, and pumpkin are rich in betacarotene.

Antioxidants: Compounds like flavonoids and polyphenols help reduce inflammation and oxidative stress, which can improve skin health. These antioxidants are abundant in a variety of fruits and vegetables.

Role of Juice Cleanses in Enhancing Skin Health

Juice cleanses provide a concentrated source of these skinfriendly nutrients, which can help support skin health and improve its appearance. The hydration provided by juices also helps maintain skin moisture and elasticity. Some ingredients like cucumbers, aloe vera, and watermelon are particularly hydrating and beneficial for the skin.

Hydration and Skin Health

Proper hydration is essential for maintaining healthy skin. When the body is wellhydrated, the skin remains supple, elastic, and less prone to dryness and wrinkles. Juices with high water content, such as those made from cucumbers, celery, and watermelon, contribute significantly to overall hydration. This increased hydration helps to flush out toxins, improve blood circulation, and keep the skin looking fresh and vibrant.

Detoxification and Skin Clarity

The skin is one of the body's largest organs and plays a significant role in detoxification. When the body is overwhelmed with toxins, it can manifest in the skin through acne, dullness, and other skin issues. Juice cleanses, which are believed to support the body's natural detox processes, can indirectly benefit skin health by helping to clear out impurities that can cause skin problems.

AntiInflammatory Benefits

Many fruits and vegetables used in juice cleanses, such as berries, leafy greens, and turmeric, have antiinflammatory properties. Chronic inflammation can contribute to various skin issues, including acne, eczema, and premature aging. By reducing inflammation, juice cleanses can help improve skin clarity and reduce the appearance of redness and puffiness.

Scientific Evidence

While there is anecdotal evidence and some research supporting the skin benefits of a nutrientrich diet, including the consumption of fruits and vegetables, specific studies on juice cleanses and skin health are limited. However, the general consensus is that a diet high in vitamins, minerals, and antioxidants supports overall skin health. Hydration and nutrient intake from juice cleanses can contribute to a temporary improvement in skin appearance, but longterm skin health is best supported by a balanced diet and consistent skincare routine.

Conclusion

Juice cleanses have garnered popularity for their potential health benefits, including detoxification, boosting immunity, improving digestion, aiding in weight loss, and enhancing skin health. While the concentrated intake of vitamins, minerals, and antioxidants can offer some immediate benefits, it's important to approach juice cleanses with a balanced perspective.

The body's natural detoxification systems, such as the liver and kidneys, are already efficient at eliminating toxins. Juice cleanses may provide a temporary boost in nutrients and hydration, supporting these processes, but they are not a substitute for the body's natural mechanisms. Similarly, while juice cleanses can lead to shortterm weight loss, primarily due to a caloric deficit and water loss, sustainable weight management requires longterm dietary and lifestyle changes.

Boosting immunity and improving digestion are benefits often associated with the high nutrient content of juices. However, the lack of fiber in juice cleanses can be a drawback for digestive health, and the direct impact on immune function needs more scientific validation.

Enhancing skin health through juice cleanses is supported by the intake of skinfriendly nutrients and increased hydration. While these can improve the skin's appearance temporarily, maintaining healthy skin over the long term involves a holistic approach, including a balanced diet, proper hydration, and a consistent skincare routine.

Ultimately, juice cleanses can be a useful tool for those seeking a shortterm nutritional boost or a reset. However, they should be approached with caution and not relied upon as a sole strategy for health and wellness. Consulting with healthcare professionals and integrating juice cleanses as part of a broader, balanced diet and healthy lifestyle is essential for achieving and maintaining optimal health.

CHAPTER 3: TYPES OF JUICE CLEANSES

OneDay Cleanse

The oneday juice cleanse is a popular choice for beginners and those looking to give their digestive system a short break. This cleanse is designed to be a gentle introduction to juice fasting, allowing individuals to experience some of the benefits of a longer cleanse without the commitment or intensity.

Benefits of a OneDay Cleanse

Digestive Rest: Even a short break from solid foods can give the digestive system time to rest and reset. This can lead to improved digestion and a reduction in bloating and discomfort.

Hydration Boost: Drinking only juices for a day can help increase overall hydration, which is beneficial for skin health, energy levels, and overall bodily functions.

Nutrient Intake: A oneday cleanse provides a concentrated dose of vitamins, minerals, and antioxidants from fruits and vegetables, which can help boost immunity and energy levels.

Mental Reset: Taking a day to focus on health and wellness can provide a mental reset, helping to reduce stress and promote mindfulness around eating habits.

How to Prepare for a OneDay Cleanse

Preparation for a oneday cleanse is relatively straightforward. It's important to start by reducing the intake of processed foods, caffeine, and alcohol a few days before the cleanse to minimize withdrawal symptoms and make the transition smoother. Increasing the intake of fruits, vegetables, and water in the days leading up to the cleanse can also help prepare the body.

Sample OneDay Cleanse Schedule

Morning: Start the day with a glass of warm lemon water to kickstart the digestive system and hydrate the body. Follow this with a green juice made from ingredients like kale, spinach, cucumber, celery, and apple.

MidMorning: A midmorning juice can include a blend of citrus fruits such as oranges, grapefruits, and lemons, which are high in vitamin C and antioxidants.

Lunch: For lunch, a more substantial juice with a mix of vegetables and a small amount of fruit can be consumed. Ingredients might include carrots, beets, apple, and ginger.

Afternoon: A hydrating juice made from ingredients like watermelon, mint, and lime can be refreshing and help maintain energy levels throughout the afternoon.

Dinner: A nutrientdense green juice similar to the morning juice can be consumed for dinner. Adding ingredients like parsley and lemon can provide additional detoxifying benefits.

Evening: Finish the day with a soothing juice made from ingredients like chamomile tea, apple, and a small amount of raw honey.

ThreeDay Cleanse

The threeday juice cleanse is one of the most popular options for those looking to experience a more thorough detoxification process. This duration allows the body to enter a deeper state of cleansing while still being manageable for most people.

Benefits of a ThreeDay Cleanse

Deeper Detoxification: A threeday cleanse provides more time for the body to eliminate toxins and reset. The extended break from solid foods allows the digestive system to rest more fully and can lead to a greater sense of rejuvenation.

Improved Energy Levels: Many people report increased energy levels and mental clarity after completing a threeday cleanse, as the body benefits from the influx of vitamins, minerals, and antioxidants.

Weight Loss: A threeday cleanse can lead to shortterm weight loss, primarily due to the reduced caloric intake and loss of water weight. It can also help kickstart healthier eating habits.

Reduced Inflammation: The antiinflammatory properties of many fruits and vegetables used in juice cleanses can help reduce inflammation in the body, which is beneficial for overall health.

How to Prepare for a ThreeDay Cleanse

Preparation for a threeday cleanse involves more extensive dietary adjustments. It's recommended to gradually eliminate processed foods, caffeine, alcohol, dairy, and meat at least three to five days before the cleanse. Increasing the intake of raw fruits and vegetables, whole grains, and plenty of water can help prepare the body for the cleanse.

Sample ThreeDay Cleanse Schedule

Day 1:

Morning: Begin with warm lemon water followed by a green juice (kale, spinach, cucumber, celery, apple).

MidMorning: A citrus blend (oranges, grapefruits, lemons).

Lunch: A hearty vegetable juice (carrots, beets, apple, ginger).

Afternoon: A hydrating juice (watermelon, mint, lime).

Dinner: A nutrientdense green juice (kale, parsley, lemon).

Evening: A soothing juice (chamomile tea, apple, raw honey).

Day 2:

Morning: Repeat the green juice.

MidMorning: A berry blend (strawberries, blueberries, raspberries, apple).

Lunch: A vegetable juice (tomatoes, celery, bell pepper, cucumber).

Afternoon: A citrus blend.

Dinner: A green juice (kale, spinach, parsley, lemon).

Evening: A calming juice (chamomile tea, apple, raw honey).

Day 3:

Morning: Start with the green juice.

MidMorning: A tropical blend (pineapple, mango, coconut water).

Lunch: A robust vegetable juice (carrots, beets, apple, ginger).

Afternoon: A hydrating juice.

Dinner: A green juice (kale, parsley, lemon).

Evening: A relaxing juice (chamomile tea, apple, raw honey).

FiveDay Cleanse

The fiveday juice cleanse is a more intensive detox program that allows for a deeper level of cleansing and rejuvenation. This cleanse is suited for those with some experience in juice fasting and who are looking for a more profound reset.

Benefits of a FiveDay Cleanse

Extended Detoxification: A fiveday cleanse provides ample time for the body to undergo significant detoxification. This can lead to a more noticeable reduction in toxins and overall improvement in health.

Enhanced Weight Loss: The extended duration can result in more substantial weight loss, which includes the loss of both water weight and fat. It can also help establish longterm healthy eating habits.

Improved Digestive Health: A fiveday break from solid foods allows the digestive system to rest and repair more thoroughly, which can lead to improved digestion and reduced symptoms of digestive distress.

Increased Mental Clarity: Many individuals report enhanced mental clarity and focus during and after a fiveday cleanse, as the body and mind benefit from the nutritional boost and reduced digestive workload.

How to Prepare for a FiveDay Cleanse

Preparing for a fiveday cleanse requires more extensive dietary changes. It's important to start eliminating processed foods, caffeine, alcohol, dairy, and meat at least five to seven days before the cleanse. Focusing on a diet rich in raw fruits, vegetables, whole grains, and plenty of water helps prepare the body for the cleanse. It's also beneficial to gradually reduce portion sizes to ease the transition to a liquidonly diet.

Sample FiveDay Cleanse Schedule

Day 1:

Morning: Warm lemon water followed by a green juice (kale, spinach, cucumber, celery, apple).

MidMorning: A citrus blend (oranges, grapefruits, lemons).

Lunch: A hearty vegetable juice (carrots, beets, apple, ginger).

Afternoon: A hydrating juice (watermelon, mint, lime).

Dinner: A nutrientdense green juice (kale, parsley, lemon).

Evening: A soothing juice (chamomile tea, apple, raw honey).

Day 2:

Morning: Repeat the green juice.

MidMorning: A berry blend (strawberries, blueberries, raspberries, apple).

Lunch: A vegetable juice (tomatoes, celery, bell pepper, cucumber).

Afternoon: A citrus blend.

Dinner: A green juice (kale, spinach, parsley, lemon).

Evening: A calming juice (chamomile tea, apple, raw honey).

Day 3:

Morning: Start with the green juice.

MidMorning: A tropical blend (pineapple, mango, coconut water).

Lunch: A robust vegetable juice (carrots, beets, apple, ginger).

Afternoon: A hydrating juice.

Dinner: A green juice (kale, parsley, lemon).

Evening: A relaxing juice (chamomile tea, apple, raw honey).

Day 4:

Morning: Green juice (kale, spinach, cucumber, celery, apple).

MidMorning: Citrus blend (oranges, grapefruits, lemons).

Lunch: Vegetable juice (carrots, beets, apple, ginger).

Afternoon: Hydrating juice (watermelon, mint, lime).

Dinner: Green juice (kale, parsley, lemon).

Evening: Soothing juice (chamomile tea, apple, raw honey).

Day 5:

Morning: Green juice.

MidMorning: Berry blend.

Lunch: Robust vegetable juice.

Afternoon: Hydrating juice.

Dinner: Green juice.

Evening: Relaxing juice.

Customizable Cleanses

Customizable juice cleanses offer flexibility and personalization, making them suitable for individuals with specific health goals, dietary preferences, or nutritional needs. These cleanses can be tailored to address particular concerns, such as weight loss, improved digestion, or enhanced skin health. Customizable cleanses allow for a more individualized approach, making it easier to adhere to the cleanse and achieve desired results.

Benefits of Customizable Cleanses

Personalization: Customizable cleanses can be tailored to meet individual health goals and dietary preferences. This personalization can lead to more effective and enjoyable cleansing experiences.

Targeted Nutrition: By selecting specific ingredients, individuals can focus on particular health concerns. For example, those looking to boost immunity might include more citrus fruits and leafy greens, while those aiming for better digestion might focus on ginger, mint, and aloe vera.

Flexibility: Customizable cleanses offer the flexibility to adjust the duration and intensity based on personal needs and lifestyle. This can make the cleanse more manageable and sustainable.

Increased Adherence: When individuals can choose ingredients they enjoy and find appealing, they are more likely to stick to the cleanse and achieve their health goals.

How to Create a Customizable Cleanse

Creating a customizable cleanse involves several steps, including setting clear health goals, selecting appropriate ingredients, and planning a schedule that fits personal preferences and lifestyle.

1. Set Clear Health Goals:
Identify the primary health goals for the cleanse, such as detoxification, weight loss, improved digestion, or enhanced skin health.

Consider any specific dietary restrictions or preferences, such as vegan, glutenfree, or lowsugar.

2. Select Appropriate Ingredients:
Choose ingredients that align with the health goals and dietary preferences. For detoxification, focus on leafy greens, citrus

fruits, and herbs like parsley and cilantro. For digestion, include ginger, mint, and aloe vera.

Ensure a balance of fruits and vegetables to provide a wide range of vitamins, minerals, and antioxidants.

3. Plan the Schedule:

Determine the duration of the cleanse based on personal goals and experience with juice fasting. Options can range from one day to several weeks.

Plan a daily schedule that includes a variety of juices to provide balanced nutrition and prevent monotony. Include a mix of green juices, fruit juices, and vegetable juices.

Sample Customizable Cleanse Schedule

Here is an example of a threeday customizable cleanse focused on detoxification and improved digestion:

Day 1:

Morning: Detox green juice (kale, spinach, cucumber, celery, lemon, parsley).

MidMorning: Citrus boost (oranges, grapefruits, lemon, mint).

Lunch: Digestion aid (carrots, beets, apple, ginger).

Afternoon: Hydration blend (watermelon, cucumber, mint).

Dinner: Cleansing green juice (kale, spinach, celery, cilantro, lemon).

Evening: Calming juice (chamomile tea, apple, raw honey).

Day 2:

Morning: Detox green juice.

MidMorning: Berry antioxidant (strawberries, blueberries, raspberries, apple).

Lunch: Vegetable blend (tomatoes, celery, bell pepper, cucumber).

Afternoon: Tropical refresh (pineapple, mango, coconut water).

Dinner: Cleansing green juice.

Evening: Relaxing juice (chamomile tea, apple, raw honey).

Day 3:
Morning: Detox green juice.
MidMorning: Citrus boost.
Lunch: Digestion aid.
Afternoon: Hydration blend.
Dinner: Cleansing green juice.
Evening: Calming juice.

Tips for Success with Customizable Cleanses

Listen to Your Body: Pay attention to how your body responds to different juices and adjust ingredients as needed. If certain juices cause discomfort or bloating, try different combinations or reduce the quantity.

Stay Hydrated: In addition to juices, drink plenty of water throughout the day to support detoxification and hydration.

Balance Fruit and Vegetable Juices: While fruit juices can be delicious, they can also be high in sugar. Balance them with vegetable juices to maintain stable blood sugar levels and provide a broader range of nutrients.

Plan for PostCleanse Transition: Gradually reintroduce solid foods after the cleanse, starting with easily digestible foods like fruits, vegetables, and whole grains. Avoid jumping straight back into processed foods or heavy meals.

Conclusion

Juice cleanses come in various forms, each with its unique benefits and considerations. The oneday cleanse is an excellent starting point for beginners, offering a gentle introduction to juice fasting and a short break for the digestive system. The threeday cleanse allows for a deeper detoxification process, providing more substantial benefits such as increased energy levels, improved digestion, and shortterm weight loss. The fiveday cleanse is a more intensive program that can lead to significant detoxification, enhanced mental clarity, and more noticeable weight loss.

Customizable cleanses offer the greatest flexibility and personalization, allowing individuals to tailor the cleanse to their specific health goals and dietary preferences. Whether the goal is detoxification, improved digestion, weight loss, or enhanced skin health, customizable cleanses provide a targeted approach to achieve desired results.

Regardless of the type of cleanse chosen, it's important to approach juice fasting with a balanced perspective. While juice cleanses can provide a concentrated source of vitamins, minerals, and antioxidants, they should not be relied upon as a sole strategy for health and wellness. A balanced diet, regular physical activity, and a healthy lifestyle are essential for longterm health and wellbeing.

Consulting with healthcare professionals before starting a juice cleanse, especially for those with underlying health conditions or dietary concerns, can ensure a safe and effective cleansing experience. By integrating juice cleanses as part of a broader, balanced diet and healthy lifestyle, individuals can enjoy the benefits of juicing while maintaining overall health and vitality.

CHAPTER 4: PREPARING FOR A JUICE CLEANSE

Preparing for a juice cleanse involves more than just stocking up on fruits and vegetables. It's about setting clear, realistic goals, gathering the right ingredients and equipment, and making dietary adjustments before you start. Proper preparation can enhance the effectiveness of the cleanse and make the experience more enjoyable and sustainable.

Setting Realistic Goals

Before embarking on a juice cleanse, it's essential to define clear, achievable goals. These goals will help guide your choices and keep you motivated throughout the cleanse.

Identify Your Reasons

Detoxification: Are you looking to give your body a break from processed foods and toxins?

Weight Loss: Is weight loss a primary goal for you?

Digestive Health: Are you seeking to improve your digestion and gut health?

Energy Boost: Do you want to increase your energy levels and mental clarity?

Skin Health: Are you aiming for clearer, more vibrant skin?

Set Achievable Objectives

Duration: Decide on the length of your cleanse. Start with a oneday cleanse if you're a beginner and gradually work up to three or five days as you become more comfortable.

Expected Outcomes: Understand that while juice cleanses can offer shortterm benefits, significant, lasting changes in weight and health require longterm lifestyle adjustments.

Health Considerations: Consider any underlying health conditions and consult with a healthcare professional to ensure a juice cleanse is safe for you.

Shopping List and Ingredients

A successful juice cleanse depends on having a wellplanned shopping list with a variety of fresh, organic fruits and vegetables. Here are some staple ingredients and their benefits:

Leafy Greens

Kale: Rich in vitamins A, C, and K, calcium, and antioxidants.

Spinach: High in iron, magnesium, and vitamins A and C.

Swiss Chard: Contains vitamins K, A, and C, and magnesium.

Fruits

Apples: Provide a natural sweetness and are high in fiber and vitamin C.

Citrus Fruits (oranges, lemons, grapefruits): Packed with vitamin C and antioxidants.

Berries (strawberries, blueberries, raspberries): Rich in antioxidants, vitamins, and fiber.

Pineapple: Contains bromelain, which aids digestion and reduces inflammation.

Vegetables

Carrots: High in betacarotene, vitamin A, and antioxidants.

Beets: Good source of iron, folate, and antioxidants.

Cucumbers: High water content for hydration and skin health.

Herbs and Spices

Ginger: Antiinflammatory and aids digestion.

Turmeric: Contains curcumin, a powerful antiinflammatory compound.

Mint: Refreshing and aids in digestion.

Parsley and Cilantro: Detoxifying and rich in vitamins.

Hydrating Ingredients

Coconut Water: Provides natural electrolytes and hydration.

Aloe Vera: Known for its digestive benefits and skin health properties.

Watermelon: High in water content and vitamins A and C.

Necessary Equipment (Juicers, Blenders)

Having the right equipment is crucial for a smooth and efficient juice cleanse. Here are some essential tools:

Juicers

Centrifugal Juicers: These are fast and affordable, making them a good option for beginners. They work by spinning fruits and vegetables at high speed to extract the juice.

Pros: Quick, easy to use, generally less expensive.

Cons: Can be noisy, produce less juice compared to other types, and may not handle leafy greens as well.

Masticating Juicers: Also known as slow or coldpress juicers, these use an auger to crush and press the produce to extract juice.

Pros: Extract more juice, especially from leafy greens, produce less foam, and preserve more nutrients due to less heat.

Cons: More expensive, slower, and typically more cumbersome to clean.

Blenders

HighSpeed Blenders: Great for making smoothies and blending whole fruits and vegetables into juices. They retain fiber, making them suitable for those who want to include more fiber in their cleanse.

Pros: Versatile, can make smoothies, soups, and other blended foods, retains fiber.

Cons: Doesn't separate juice from pulp, resulting in thicker drinks.

Regular Blenders: Suitable for basic blending needs but may struggle with tougher ingredients like leafy greens and dense vegetables.

Additional Tools

Strainers or Nut Milk Bags: Useful for straining blended juices to remove pulp if a smoother texture is desired.

Mason Jars or Glass Bottles: Ideal for storing freshly made juices and taking them on the go.

Cutting Boards and Knives: Highquality, sharp knives and sturdy cutting boards will make the preparation process faster and safer.

PreCleanse Diet Tips

Preparing your body for a juice cleanse is essential to minimize detox symptoms and ensure a smooth transition. Here are some tips:

Gradually Eliminate Certain Foods

Processed Foods and Sugars: Start reducing your intake of processed foods, refined sugars, and artificial sweeteners at least a week before the cleanse.

Caffeine and Alcohol: Gradually cut back on caffeine and alcohol to prevent withdrawal symptoms such as headaches and fatigue.

Dairy and Meat: Begin to limit dairy and meat consumption, focusing more on plantbased foods.

Increase Fresh Produce Intake

Fruits and Vegetables: Start incorporating more raw and cooked fruits and vegetables into your diet. This helps increase your fiber intake and prepares your digestive system for the cleanse.

Whole Grains: Include whole grains like quinoa, brown rice, and oats to provide sustained energy and fiber.

Stay Hydrated

Water: Drink plenty of water throughout the day to stay hydrated and support your body's natural detoxification processes.

Herbal Teas: Incorporate herbal teas such as chamomile, peppermint, and ginger tea, which can aid digestion and provide a soothing effect.

Balanced Meals

Smaller, Frequent Meals: Eat smaller, more frequent meals to prevent overeating and ease the digestive workload.

Balanced Nutrition: Ensure your meals are balanced with a mix of carbohydrates, proteins, and healthy fats. This will help maintain your energy levels and reduce cravings.

Listen to Your Body

Rest: Ensure you're getting enough rest and sleep, as your body will be working to detoxify and heal.

Mindfulness: Practice mindful eating, paying attention to how your body feels and making conscious choices about what you eat.

Example PreCleanse Diet Plan

Day 12:

Breakfast: Smoothie with spinach, banana, almond milk, and chia seeds.

Snack: Apple with a handful of almonds.

Lunch: Salad with mixed greens, cherry tomatoes, cucumbers, quinoa, and olive oil dressing.

Snack: Carrot sticks with hummus.

Dinner: Steamed vegetables with brown rice and a squeeze of lemon.

Day 34:

Breakfast: Oatmeal with berries and a drizzle of honey.

Snack: Sliced cucumber and bell peppers.

Lunch: Lentil soup with a side salad.

Snack: Fresh fruit (e.g., orange or pear).

Dinner: Baked sweet potato with steamed broccoli and a sprinkle of sea salt.

Day 56:

Breakfast: Fresh fruit salad with a squeeze of lime.

Snack: Green smoothie with kale, pineapple, and coconut water.

Lunch: Veggie wrap with avocado, sprouts, and mixed greens.

Snack: Sliced mango or watermelon.

Dinner: Stirfried vegetables with tofu and a light soy sauce.

By setting realistic goals, gathering the necessary ingredients and equipment, and following a precleanse diet, you can ensure a successful and enjoyable juice cleanse experience. Proper preparation will help your body adjust to the cleanse more smoothly, reduce potential detox symptoms, and enhance the overall benefits. Remember, the key to a successful juice cleanse is listening to your body and making adjustments as needed to suit your individual needs and preferences.

CHAPTER 5: JUICE CLEANSE RECIPES

Juice cleanses are a popular way to detoxify the body, boost immunity, improve digestion, and enhance overall health. They involve consuming only juices made from fresh fruits and vegetables for a set period, allowing the body to rest from digesting solid foods. Here, we provide detailed recipes for five different juices that can be part of a juice cleanse: Green Detox Juice, Citrus Immunity Booster, Berry Antioxidant Blend, Refreshing Hydration Mix, and ProteinPacked Vegetable Juice. Each recipe is designed to offer unique health benefits and can be easily made at home with a juicer or blender.

Green Detox Juice

Ingredients:

1 cucumber

2 celery stalks

1 handful of spinach

1 handful of kale

1 green apple

1 lemon

1inch piece of ginger

Benefits:

Cucumber: Hydrating and cooling, cucumbers are low in calories but high in vitamins and minerals, including vitamin K.

Celery: Known for its antiinflammatory properties, celery is also rich in vitamins A, C, and K.

Spinach and Kale: These leafy greens are nutrient powerhouses, packed with vitamins A, C, K, and folate, as well as iron and calcium.

Green Apple: Adds a touch of sweetness and is high in fiber and vitamin C.

Lemon: Aids digestion and detoxification, and is high in vitamin C.

Ginger: Antiinflammatory and aids digestion.

Instructions:

1. Wash all the ingredients thoroughly.

2. Peel the lemon and ginger.

3. Cut the cucumber, celery, green apple, and ginger into smaller pieces if needed to fit your juicer or blender.

4. Juice all the ingredients together. If using a blender, blend the ingredients with a little water and strain through a fine mesh strainer or nut milk bag to remove the pulp.

5. Stir well and serve immediately for the best taste and nutrient retention.

Nutritional Information:

This juice is rich in vitamins A, C, and K, and provides a good dose of iron and antioxidants. It is low in calories and can help in detoxifying the liver and promoting overall health.

Citrus Immunity Booster

Ingredients:

2 oranges
1 grapefruit
1 lemon
1 small piece of turmeric root (or 1/2 teaspoon turmeric powder)
1 small piece of ginger

Benefits:

Oranges and Grapefruit: High in vitamin C, which is essential for immune function and skin health. They also contain antioxidants like flavonoids.

Lemon: Enhances detoxification and provides additional vitamin C.

Turmeric: Contains curcumin, a powerful antiinflammatory compound that boosts immune function.

Ginger: Antiinflammatory and promotes healthy digestion.

Instructions:

1. Wash all the ingredients thoroughly.
2. Peel the oranges, grapefruit, lemon, turmeric, and ginger.
3. Cut the fruits and roots into smaller pieces to fit your juicer or blender.
4. Juice all the ingredients together. If using a blender, blend the ingredients with a little water and strain to remove the pulp.
5. Stir well and serve immediately.

Nutritional Information:

This juice is a powerhouse of vitamin C and antioxidants. It helps boost the immune system, reduce inflammation, and support overall health. The citrus fruits also provide a refreshing and tangy flavor.

Berry Antioxidant Blend

Ingredients:

1 cup strawberries
1 cup blueberries
1 cup raspberries
1 apple
1 handful of spinach
1 tablespoon chia seeds (optional)

Benefits:

Berries (Strawberries, Blueberries, Raspberries): Packed with antioxidants, vitamins, and fiber, berries help fight free radicals and reduce inflammation.

Apple: Adds sweetness and provides fiber and vitamin C.

Spinach: Adds extra nutrients, including vitamins A, C, K, and iron.

Chia Seeds: High in omega3 fatty acids, fiber, and protein, chia seeds can be added for an extra nutritional boost.

Instructions:

1. Wash all the ingredients thoroughly.
2. Remove the stems from the strawberries.
3. Core the apple and cut it into smaller pieces.
4. Juice the berries, apple, and spinach together. If using a blender, blend the ingredients with a little water and strain to remove the pulp.

5. Stir in the chia seeds (if using) and let the juice sit for a few minutes to allow the seeds to swell.

6. Serve immediately.

Nutritional Information:

This juice is high in antioxidants, particularly vitamin C and anthocyanins from the berries. It also provides fiber, iron, and other essential nutrients, making it excellent for overall health and skin vitality.

Refreshing Hydration Mix

Ingredients:

1 cucumber

1 cup watermelon

1 lime

1 handful of mint leaves

1/2 cup coconut water

Benefits:

Cucumber: Hydrating and cooling, providing vitamins K and C.

Watermelon: High in water content and contains vitamins A, C, and antioxidants like lycopene.

Lime: Adds a zesty flavor and is high in vitamin C.

Mint: Refreshing and aids in digestion.

Coconut Water: Natural electrolytes make it excellent for hydration.

Instructions:

1. Wash all the ingredients thoroughly.
2. Peel the lime.
3. Cut the cucumber and watermelon into smaller pieces.

4. Juice the cucumber, watermelon, lime, and mint leaves together. If using a blender, blend the ingredients with a little water and strain to remove the pulp.

5. Mix in the coconut water.

6. Stir well and serve immediately.

Nutritional Information:

This juice is incredibly hydrating and refreshing, perfect for hot days or after a workout. It provides a good mix of vitamins and minerals, including vitamin C, potassium, and antioxidants.

ProteinPacked Vegetable Juice

Ingredients:

2 carrots

2 celery stalks

1 red bell pepper

1 handful of spinach

1 tomato

1/2 avocado

1 tablespoon hemp seeds (optional)

Benefits:

Carrots: High in betacarotene, vitamin A, and antioxidants.

Celery: Antiinflammatory and rich in vitamins A, C, and K.

Red Bell Pepper: Contains high amounts of vitamin C, antioxidants, and fiber.

Spinach: Packed with vitamins A, C, K, iron, and protein.

Tomato: Rich in lycopene, vitamins A and C, and potassium.

Avocado: Provides healthy fats, fiber, and a small amount of protein.

Hemp Seeds: High in protein, omega3 and omega6 fatty acids, and other essential nutrients.

Instructions:

1. Wash all the ingredients thoroughly.
2. Peel the carrots if not using organic.
3. Cut the carrots, celery, bell pepper, and tomato into smaller pieces.
4. Juice the carrots, celery, bell pepper, spinach, and tomato together. If using a blender, blend the ingredients with a little water and strain to remove the pulp.
5. Blend in the avocado until smooth. If using hemp seeds, stir them into the juice.
6. Serve immediately.

Nutritional Information:

This juice is rich in vitamins A, C, and K, and provides a good amount of protein and healthy fats from the avocado and hemp seeds. It's a great option for those looking to increase their vegetable intake and support muscle repair and growth.

Conclusion

Juice cleanses offer a convenient and delicious way to boost your intake of essential nutrients, support detoxification, and improve overall health. These five juice recipes—Green Detox Juice, Citrus Immunity Booster, Berry Antioxidant Blend, Refreshing Hydration Mix, and ProteinPacked Vegetable Juice—each provide unique health benefits and can be easily incorporated into a juice cleanse regimen.

When preparing these juices, always use fresh, organic ingredients whenever possible to maximize the nutritional content and minimize exposure to pesticides and other harmful chemicals. Proper preparation and equipment are key to making the process smooth and enjoyable.

Remember, while juice cleanses can offer many benefits, they should be part of a balanced and healthy lifestyle. Listen to your body, consult with a healthcare professional if you have any underlying health conditions, and enjoy the journey to better health and wellness.

CHAPTER 6: DURING THE CLEANSE

Successfully navigating a juice cleanse requires a structured daily schedule, strategies for managing hunger and cravings, staying hydrated, and monitoring your body's responses. This section provides a comprehensive guide to help you through the process, ensuring you get the most out of your cleanse while maintaining your wellbeing.

Daily Schedule and Routine

Establishing a daily schedule can provide structure and support during your juice cleanse. Here is an example of a daily routine to follow:

Morning:

7:00 AM: Start your day with a glass of warm water with lemon. This helps kickstart your metabolism and begin the detoxification process.

8:00 AM: Drink your first juice of the day. A green detox juice is a great choice to provide essential nutrients and antioxidants.

MidMorning:

10:00 AM: Drink a second juice, such as the Citrus Immunity Booster, to keep your energy levels up and support your immune system.

Lunch:

12:00 PM: Have a third juice, like the Berry Antioxidant Blend, to sustain your energy and provide a rich source of vitamins and antioxidants.

Afternoon:

2:00 PM: Drink another juice, such as the Refreshing Hydration Mix, to stay hydrated and refreshed.

4:00 PM: Enjoy a fifth juice, like a ProteinPacked Vegetable Juice, to provide essential nutrients and help you feel full.

Evening:

6:00 PM: Have your final juice of the day. Choose a calming and nourishing juice, such as a green detox juice or a hydration mix.

8:00 PM: Drink a cup of herbal tea, such as chamomile or peppermint, to help relax and prepare for a restful night.

Tips for Maintaining Your Schedule:

Consistency: Try to stick to the same schedule each day to help your body adjust to the routine.

Preparation: Make your juices in advance to save time and ensure you stay on track.

Listen to Your Body: If you feel hungry or fatigued, adjust the timing of your juices as needed. It's important to nourish your body adequately.

Managing Hunger and Cravings

Hunger and cravings are common challenges during a juice cleanse. Here are some strategies to help manage them:

Stay Hydrated:

Drink plenty of water throughout the day. Sometimes, thirst can be mistaken for hunger.

Herbal teas can also provide hydration and a comforting routine.

Distraction Techniques:

Engage in activities that keep your mind and body occupied, such as reading, walking, or gentle yoga.
Practice mindfulness and meditation to help manage cravings and stay focused on your goals.

Opt for FiberRich Juices:

Include juices with higher fiber content, such as those made with apples, berries, and leafy greens. Fiber can help you feel fuller for longer.

Chew Your Juices:

Swish your juices around in your mouth before swallowing. This can help stimulate digestion and make you feel more satisfied.

Healthy Snacking:

If you find it difficult to manage hunger, consider incorporating small, healthy snacks such as cucumber slices, celery sticks, or a handful of nuts. Choose snacks that align with the cleanse principles.

Mental Strategies:

Remind yourself of your goals and the reasons for doing the cleanse. Keeping a journal can help track your progress and maintain motivation.
Visualize the benefits you hope to achieve, such as improved energy levels, better digestion, and clearer skin.

Staying Hydrated

Proper hydration is crucial during a juice cleanse. Here's how to ensure you stay adequately hydrated:

Water Intake:

Aim to drink at least 810 glasses of water daily, in addition to your juices. This helps flush out toxins and keeps your body functioning optimally.

Carry a water bottle with you to remind yourself to drink water throughout the day.

Hydrating Juices:

Include hydrating ingredients in your juices, such as cucumber, watermelon, and coconut water. These not only provide hydration but also essential electrolytes.

Herbal Teas:

Herbal teas can be a soothing way to stay hydrated. Choose caffeinefree options like chamomile, peppermint, or ginger tea. These can also aid in digestion and relaxation.

Electrolyte Balance:

Consider adding a pinch of sea salt or Himalayan salt to your juices to help maintain electrolyte balance, especially if you're sweating or exercising.

Monitoring Your Body's Responses

During a juice cleanse, it's important to pay attention to how your body responds. This can help you make adjustments and ensure a safe and effective cleanse.

Common Detox Symptoms:

Headaches: Often caused by caffeine withdrawal or detoxification. Drink plenty of water and rest if needed.

Fatigue: A common symptom as your body adjusts to the cleanse. Ensure you get enough rest and consider taking short naps if necessary.

Digestive Changes: You might experience changes in bowel movements, such as increased frequency or looser stools. This is usually temporary and part of the detox process.

Positive Signs:

Increased Energy: Many people report feeling more energetic after the initial detox phase.

Improved Digestion: Your digestive system may feel lighter and more efficient.

Clearer Skin: As your body detoxifies, you may notice improvements in your skin's appearance.

When to Be Concerned:

Severe Fatigue or Weakness: If you feel excessively tired or weak, consider adjusting the cleanse or incorporating small meals.

Dizziness or Lightheadedness: These can be signs of low blood sugar or dehydration. Drink more fluids and consider eating a small, healthy snack.

Persistent Symptoms: If any symptoms persist or worsen, consult with a healthcare professional to ensure there are no underlying health issues.

Keeping a Journal:

Track your daily intake of juices and water.

Note any symptoms or changes in how you feel.

Reflect on your emotional and mental state throughout the cleanse.

Listen to Your Body:

Everyone's experience with a juice cleanse is different. What works for one person may not work for another. Be flexible and willing to adjust your cleanse as needed.

PostCleanse Transition:

Plan for a gradual transition back to solid foods after the cleanse. Start with light, easily digestible foods like fruits, vegetables, and whole grains.

Avoid jumping straight back into processed foods or heavy meals, as this can shock your digestive system.

Conclusion

Navigating a juice cleanse requires careful planning and mindfulness. By establishing a daily schedule, managing hunger and cravings, staying hydrated, and monitoring your body's responses, you can ensure a successful and beneficial cleanse. Remember that the primary goal of a juice cleanse is to support your overall health and wellbeing, so it's important to listen to your body and make adjustments as needed. A wellexecuted juice cleanse can leave you feeling rejuvenated, energized, and ready to maintain healthier habits in the long term.

CHAPTER 7: POSTCLEANSE: TRANSITIONING BACK TO SOLID FOODS

Completing a juice cleanse is an accomplishment, but it's just as important to transition back to solid foods properly to maintain the benefits and avoid any digestive discomfort. This section provides a guide on how to gradually reintroduce solid foods, maintain the benefits of the cleanse, and establish longterm healthy eating habits.

Gradual Reintroduction of Solid Foods

After a juice cleanse, your digestive system may be more sensitive, so it's crucial to reintroduce solid foods gradually and thoughtfully. Here's a stepbystep approach to ensure a smooth transition:

Day 12: Light and EasytoDigest Foods

Start with light, easytodigest foods to ease your digestive system back into processing solid foods.

Morning: Begin with a smoothie made from fruits and vegetables. You can add a small amount of almond milk or water for consistency.

MidMorning Snack: Fresh fruit like apples, pears, or berries.

Lunch: A simple vegetable soup or brothbased soup with soft, cooked vegetables.

Afternoon Snack: Raw vegetable sticks (such as cucumber or carrots) or a small handful of nuts.

Dinner: A salad with leafy greens, cucumbers, and a light vinaigrette. Avoid heavy dressings or toppings.

Day 34: Adding More Variety

Gradually introduce more variety and slightly more complex foods.

Morning: A bowl of oatmeal with fresh fruits and a sprinkle of nuts or seeds.

MidMorning Snack: A small piece of whole fruit or a handful of raw nuts.

Lunch: A larger salad with a variety of vegetables and a light protein source such as chickpeas or quinoa.

Afternoon Snack: A piece of fruit or vegetable sticks with hummus.

Dinner: A light meal with steamed or roasted vegetables and a small portion of lean protein like tofu or fish.

Day 57: Incorporating Regular Meals

Begin to reintroduce regular meals, keeping them balanced and nutritious.

Morning: Smoothie or oatmeal with added fruits, nuts, and seeds.

MidMorning Snack: Fresh fruit or a small serving of yogurt with berries.

Lunch: A hearty salad with mixed greens, vegetables, a protein source (like grilled chicken or beans), and a healthy fat source (like avocado or nuts).

Afternoon Snack: Vegetable sticks with hummus or a small handful of nuts.

Dinner: A balanced meal with lean protein, whole grains (like quinoa or brown rice), and a variety of cooked vegetables.

Day 8 and Beyond: Balanced Diet

Return to a balanced diet, focusing on whole, minimally processed foods.

Morning: Continue with smoothies, oatmeal, or other healthy breakfast options.

MidMorning Snack: Fresh fruit, nuts, or seeds.

Lunch: Balanced meals with a variety of vegetables, whole grains, and proteins.

Afternoon Snack: Fresh fruit, nuts, vegetable sticks, or yogurt.

Dinner: A balanced meal similar to lunch, incorporating different proteins, grains, and vegetables.

Maintaining Benefits of the Cleanse

To maintain the benefits of the cleanse, it's essential to continue healthy eating habits and lifestyle practices. Here are some tips:

Continue Hydrating:

Drink plenty of water throughout the day to stay hydrated and support your body's detoxification processes.

Include herbal teas and waterrich foods like fruits and vegetables.

Prioritize Whole Foods:

Focus on whole, minimally processed foods, such as fresh fruits, vegetables, whole grains, lean proteins, nuts, and seeds.
Avoid processed foods, refined sugars, and artificial ingredients.

Balanced Meals:

Ensure your meals are balanced with a good mix of macronutrients—carbohydrates, proteins, and healthy fats.
Incorporate a variety of colorful fruits and vegetables to get a wide range of nutrients.

Mindful Eating:

Practice mindful eating by paying attention to your hunger and fullness cues.

Chew your food thoroughly and savor each bite to enhance digestion and satisfaction.

Regular Physical Activity:

Incorporate regular physical activity into your routine, such as walking, yoga, or strength training.

Exercise helps maintain energy levels, supports digestion, and promotes overall wellbeing.

Stress Management:

Practice stress management techniques like meditation, deep breathing exercises, or spending time in nature.

Reducing stress supports your body's ability to maintain the benefits of the cleanse.

LongTerm Healthy Eating Habits

Establishing longterm healthy eating habits is key to sustaining the benefits of your juice cleanse and promoting overall health and wellbeing. Here are some strategies to help you maintain a healthy diet:

Meal Planning and Preparation:

Plan your meals ahead of time to ensure you have healthy options available.
Prepare meals and snacks in advance to avoid the temptation of unhealthy choices.

Healthy Cooking Methods:

Choose healthy cooking methods such as steaming, grilling, roasting, or baking.
Avoid deepfrying or using excessive amounts of unhealthy fats and oils.

Portion Control:

Be mindful of portion sizes to avoid overeating.
Use smaller plates and bowls to help control portion sizes and prevent mindless eating.

Incorporate Variety:

Include a wide variety of foods in your diet to ensure you get all the necessary nutrients.
Experiment with new fruits, vegetables, grains, and proteins to keep your meals interesting and nutritious.

Listen to Your Body:

Pay attention to how different foods make you feel and adjust your diet accordingly.
Avoid foods that cause discomfort or digestive issues.

Healthy Snacking:

Keep healthy snacks on hand, such as fresh fruits, vegetable sticks, nuts, and seeds.
Avoid processed snacks high in sugar, salt, and unhealthy fats.

Mindful Indulgence:

Allow yourself occasional treats in moderation to avoid feelings of deprivation.
Choose healthier alternatives for indulgent foods, such as dark chocolate or homemade treats with natural sweeteners.

Stay Educated:

Continuously educate yourself about nutrition and healthy eating habits.
Stay informed about new research and dietary recommendations to make informed choices.

Support System:

Surround yourself with a supportive network of friends, family, or a community focused on healthy living.
Share recipes, tips, and experiences to stay motivated and inspired.

Example PostCleanse Meal Plan

Here's an example of a balanced, healthy meal plan to follow after your juice cleanse:

Day 1:

Breakfast: Smoothie with spinach, banana, almond milk, and chia seeds.
Snack: Apple slices with almond butter.
Lunch: Quinoa salad with mixed greens, cherry tomatoes, cucumber, and a lemon vinaigrette.

Snack: Carrot sticks with hummus.

Dinner: Grilled salmon with steamed broccoli and brown rice.

Day 2:

Breakfast: Overnight oats with berries, nuts, and a drizzle of honey.

Snack: A handful of mixed nuts.

Lunch: Lentil soup with a side salad.

Snack: Fresh fruit, such as an orange or pear.

Dinner: Stirfried vegetables with tofu and quinoa.

Day 3:

Breakfast: Greek yogurt with granola and fresh fruit.

Snack: Celery sticks with peanut butter.

Lunch: Whole grain wrap with avocado, sprouts, mixed greens, and a light dressing.

Snack: A small smoothie with berries and almond milk.

Dinner: Baked chicken breast with roasted sweet potatoes and green beans.

By following a structured approach to reintroducing solid foods, maintaining the benefits of the cleanse, and establishing longterm healthy eating habits, you can sustain the positive effects of your juice cleanse and promote overall health and wellbeing. Remember, the key to lasting success is consistency and making mindful choices that support your health goals.

CHAPTER 8: POTENTIAL RISKS AND CONSIDERATIONS

Embarking on a juice cleanse can offer various health benefits, but it's essential to understand the potential risks, who should avoid juice cleanses, common side effects, and the importance of consulting with healthcare professionals before starting.

Who Should Avoid Juice Cleanses

While juice cleanses can be beneficial for many people, there are certain groups who should avoid them or proceed with caution:

1. Pregnant or Nursing Women: During pregnancy and breastfeeding, it's crucial to maintain a balanced diet that provides essential nutrients for both the mother and baby. Juice cleanses may not provide adequate calories, protein, and nutrients needed during these stages.

2. Children and Adolescents: Young individuals have specific nutritional needs for growth and development. Juice cleanses may not provide sufficient calories, protein, and other essential nutrients needed for their growth.

3. Individuals with Certain Medical Conditions: People with diabetes, kidney disease, liver disease, or other chronic health conditions should avoid juice cleanses or consult with a healthcare professional before starting. Juice cleanses can affect blood sugar levels, electrolyte balance, and medication effectiveness.

4. People with Eating Disorders:
Individuals with a history of eating disorders or disordered eating patterns should avoid restrictive diets like juice cleanses. These diets can reinforce unhealthy behaviors and disrupt normal eating patterns.

5. Individuals with Low Blood Pressure:
Juice cleanses, especially those low in sodium, can cause a drop in blood pressure, leading to dizziness, lightheadedness, or fainting.

6. People Taking Certain Medications:
Some medications may interact with the nutrients in juices or be less effective when taken on an empty stomach. It's essential to consult with a healthcare provider to ensure safety.

Common Side Effects and How to Mitigate Them

Juice cleanses can trigger various side effects as the body adjusts to a liquid diet and detoxification process. Here are some common side effects and strategies to mitigate them:

1. Hunger and Food Cravings:

Mitigation: Stay hydrated with water and herbal teas. Choose juices with higher fiber content or add nut milk for more satiety. Engage in light activities to distract from cravings.

2. Fatigue and Weakness:

Mitigation: Ensure you're drinking enough juices to meet your calorie needs. Take short naps or rest as needed. Gradually reintroduce solid foods to replenish energy stores.

3. Headaches:

Mitigation: Drink plenty of water to stay hydrated. Gradually reduce caffeine intake before starting the cleanse. If headaches persist, consider adding a small amount of caffeine through green tea or herbal teas.

4. Digestive Issues (Bloating, Diarrhea, Constipation):

Mitigation: Start with juices that are easier to digest, such as those with less fiber. Drink plenty of water to support digestion. Add probiotics or fermented foods to your diet postcleanse to promote gut health.

5. Changes in Mood or Irritability:

Mitigation: Practice relaxation techniques like yoga or meditation. Ensure you're getting enough calories and nutrients from your juices.

6. Muscle Loss:

Mitigation: Include juices with proteinrich ingredients like nuts, seeds, or nut butter.

Consider adding small amounts of plantbased protein powder if needed.

Consulting with Healthcare Professionals

Before starting a juice cleanse, it's crucial to consult with a healthcare professional, especially if you have underlying health conditions or are taking medications. Here's why it's important:

1. **Personalized Assessment:** A healthcare provider can assess your overall health, medical history, and nutritional needs to determine if a juice cleanse is suitable for you.

2. **Monitoring:** Healthcare professionals can monitor your progress during and after the cleanse, ensuring it's safe and effective for your specific health needs.

3. Medication Considerations: Some medications may need to be adjusted or taken with food, which may not be compatible with a juice cleanse. Your healthcare provider can provide guidance on medication management during the cleanse.

4. Nutritional Guidance: Healthcare professionals can offer personalized nutritional advice to help you get the most out of your cleanse while meeting your body's needs for essential nutrients.

5. Safety Precautions: They can advise on potential risks and help you mitigate side effects to ensure a safe cleansing experience.

Conclusion

While juice cleanses can offer benefits such as detoxification, weight loss, and improved digestion, they are not suitable for everyone. Understanding the potential risks, who should avoid juice cleanses, common side effects, and the importance of consulting with healthcare professionals is essential before starting any cleanse. By taking these considerations into account, you can make an informed decision about whether a juice cleanse is right for you and ensure a safe and beneficial experience for your overall health and wellbeing.

CHAPTER 9: SUCCESS STORIES AND TESTIMONIALS

Exploring success stories and testimonials from individuals who have undergone juice cleanses can provide valuable insights, motivation, and practical tips for those considering or currently undertaking a cleanse.

RealLife Experiences

Case Study: Sarah's Transformation

Sarah, a 35yearold office manager, embarked on a fiveday juice cleanse to kickstart her journey towards a healthier lifestyle. Here's her experience:

Motivation: Sarah decided to try a juice cleanse after feeling sluggish and noticing her energy levels were low. She wanted to detoxify her body and reset her eating habits.

Preparation: Leading up to the cleanse, Sarah researched different juice recipes and invested in a highquality juicer. She also stocked up on fresh produce and herbal teas to support her cleanse.

Daily Routine: During the cleanse, Sarah followed a structured daily routine. She started her mornings with warm lemon water and followed with a variety of homemade juices throughout the day. Her favorite was a green detox juice made with kale, spinach, cucumber, celery, and a hint of lemon.

Challenges: Sarah initially struggled with mild headaches and cravings for solid foods, especially during the first two days. However, she stayed motivated by reminding herself of her goals and engaging in light activities like yoga and walks in nature.

Results: By the end of the cleanse, Sarah reported feeling lighter, more energetic, and mentally clear. She noticed improvements in her digestion and skin complexion. Sarah was inspired to continue incorporating fresh juices and whole foods into her daily diet.

Reflection: Reflecting on her experience, Sarah emphasized the importance of listening to her body's signals and staying committed to her goals. She plans to incorporate regular juice days into her monthly routine to maintain the benefits of the cleanse.

Tips from Juice Cleanse Veterans

Tip 1: Prepare Mentally and Physically

Advice: "Prepare yourself mentally and physically before starting a juice cleanse. Set clear goals and understand why you're doing it. Stock up on fresh fruits and vegetables, and invest in a good juicer."

Tip 2: Stay Hydrated and Rested

Advice: "Drink plenty of water throughout the day to stay hydrated. Take short naps or rest as needed, especially during the first few days when your body is adjusting."

Tip 3: Listen to Your Body

Advice: "Listen to your body's signals. If you feel excessively tired or weak, consider adjusting your cleanse or incorporating small, nutritious snacks. Don't push yourself too hard."

Tip 4: Engage in Light Activities

Advice: "Stay active but avoid intense workouts during a cleanse. Gentle activities like yoga, walks, or stretching can help maintain energy levels and reduce stress."

Tip 5: PostCleanse Transition

Advice: "Plan your postcleanse meals wisely. Start with light, easytodigest foods and gradually reintroduce solid foods. Focus on whole, nutrientdense foods to maintain the benefits of your cleanse."

Tip 6: Journal Your Experience

Advice: "Keep a journal to track your progress, jot down how you feel each day, and note any insights or challenges. It can be motivating to see your journey unfold on paper."

Conclusion

Success stories and tips from juice cleanse veterans offer valuable guidance and encouragement for individuals considering or currently undertaking a cleanse. Reallife experiences like Sarah's demonstrate the transformative effects of a wellplanned cleanse, while veteran tips provide practical advice on preparation, hydration, listening to your body, engaging in light activities, transitioning postcleanse, and documenting your journey. By learning from these experiences and tips, you can navigate your own cleanse journey effectively, maximize benefits, and maintain a healthier lifestyle in the long term.

CHAPTER 10: FAQs ABOUT JUICE CLEANSES

Addressing common questions and concerns about juice cleanses can help individuals make informed decisions and understand what to expect during and after the cleanse process.

What is a Juice Cleanse?

A juice cleanse, also known as a juice fast or detox diet, involves consuming only fruit and vegetable juices for a certain period. The goal is to detoxify the body, promote weight loss, and improve overall health by eliminating solid foods and providing concentrated nutrients.

Are Juice Cleanses Safe?

Juice cleanses can be safe for most people when done correctly and for short periods. However, they may not be suitable for everyone, especially pregnant or nursing women, children, individuals with certain medical conditions, and those with a history of eating disorders. Consulting with a healthcare professional before starting a cleanse is recommended.

What are the Benefits of a Juice Cleanse?

Juice cleanses are believed to offer several benefits, including:

Detoxification: Eliminating toxins from the body and supporting liver function.

Weight Loss: Temporary weight loss due to reduced calorie intake.

Improved Digestion: Resting the digestive system and potentially alleviating bloating or digestive discomfort.

Increased Energy: Providing concentrated vitamins, minerals, and antioxidants that may boost energy levels.

Enhanced Skin Health: Clearer skin due to reduced intake of processed foods and potential hydration benefits from juices.

How Long Should a Juice Cleanse Last?

The duration of a juice cleanse can vary depending on individual goals and preferences. Common durations include oneday, threeday, fiveday, or even longer cleanses. It's essential to listen to your body and consult with a healthcare professional to determine a suitable duration.

What Should I Expect During a Juice Cleanse?

During a juice cleanse, you may experience various effects as your body adjusts to the liquid diet and detoxification process. Common experiences include:

Hunger and Food Cravings: Especially in the initial days of the cleanse.

Increased Urination: As the body eliminates toxins and excess fluids.

Mild Detox Symptoms: Such as headaches, fatigue, or digestive changes.

Improved Energy and Clarity: Reported by some individuals as the cleanse progresses.

How Do I Prepare for a Juice Cleanse?

Preparing for a juice cleanse involves several steps:

Research: Learn about different cleanse options, juice recipes, and potential benefits.

Shopping: Stock up on fresh fruits, vegetables, and other cleansefriendly ingredients.

Equipment: Invest in a quality juicer or blender if necessary.

Consultation: Consider consulting with a healthcare professional, especially if you have underlying health conditions or concerns.

What Should I Drink During a Juice Cleanse?

During a juice cleanse, you should primarily drink freshly made fruit and vegetable juices. Popular options include green juices (kale, spinach, cucumber), citrus juices (lemon, orange), and antioxidantrich juices (berries, carrots). It's essential to drink plenty of water and herbal teas to stay hydrated.

How Do I Break a Juice Cleanse?

Breaking a juice cleanse is crucial to avoid digestive discomfort and maintain the benefits of the cleanse. Gradually reintroduce solid foods over several days, starting with light, easily digestible foods like smoothies, soups, and salads. Avoid processed foods, heavy meals, and excessive caffeine or alcohol immediately postcleanse.

Can I Exercise During a Juice Cleanse?

Light exercise like walking, yoga, or stretching is generally recommended during a juice cleanse to support circulation, metabolism, and overall wellbeing. Avoid intense workouts or activities that require significant energy expenditure, as your calorie intake will be reduced during the cleanse.

How Often Can I Do a Juice Cleanse?

The frequency of juice cleanses depends on individual health goals and preferences. Some people may do a cleanse once a month or as a seasonal detox, while others may incorporate occasional juice days into their routine. It's essential to listen to your body and consult with a healthcare professional to determine a safe and sustainable approach.

In conclusion, understanding the basics of juice cleanses, including their benefits, safety considerations, preparation tips, and what to expect during and after the cleanse, can help individuals make informed decisions about incorporating this dietary practice into their lifestyle. By addressing common questions and concerns through FAQs, individuals can navigate their cleanse experience effectively and maximize potential benefits for overall health and wellbeing. Always prioritize your health and consult with a healthcare professional before starting any new diet or cleanse regimen.

RESOURCES AND FURTHER READING

Exploring resources and further reading can provide additional information, guidance, and support for individuals interested in juice cleanses. Here are recommended books and articles, online communities and support groups, as well as additional recipes and meal plans to enhance your cleanse experience.

Recommended Books and Articles

1. Books:

The Juice Cleanse Reset Diet by Lori Kenyon Farley and Marra St. Clair

The Big Book of Juices by Natalie Savona

Juice Fasting and Detoxification by Steve Meyerowitz

2. Articles:

"The Truth About Juice Cleanses" Harvard Health Publishing

"Juice Cleanse: The Pros, Cons, and Tips for Success" WebMD

"Are Juice Cleanses Healthy? Benefits and Risks" Healthline

Online Communities and Support Groups

Joining online communities and support groups can provide motivation, tips, and shared experiences throughout your juice cleanse journey. Here are some platforms to consider:

Reddit Communities: Explore subreddits like r/Juicing and r/DetoxDiets for discussions, recipes, and support from fellow cleanse enthusiasts.

Facebook Groups: Join groups such as "Juice Cleanse Support Group" or "Juice Detox and Cleansing Recipes" for community support and recipe ideas.

Instagram: Follow hashtags like JuiceCleanse and DetoxDiet for inspiration and reallife testimonials from individuals sharing their cleanse experiences.

Additional Recipes and Meal Plans

Expand your juice cleanse repertoire with additional recipes and meal plans designed to support your cleanse goals:

1. Recipes:

Green Detox Juice: Kale, spinach, cucumber, celery, green apple, lemon.

Citrus Immunity Booster: Oranges, grapefruits, lemon, ginger.

Berry Antioxidant Blend: Blueberries, strawberries, raspberries, spinach, almond milk.

Refreshing Hydration Mix: Cucumber, mint, watermelon, coconut water.

ProteinPacked Vegetable Juice: Carrots, beets, celery, parsley, pea protein powder.

2. Sample Meal Plans:

Day 1:
Breakfast: Green Detox Juice
Snack: Berry Antioxidant Blend
Lunch: ProteinPacked Vegetable Juice
Snack: Citrus Immunity Booster
Dinner: Refreshing Hydration Mix

Day 2:
Breakfast: Citrus Immunity Booster
Snack: ProteinPacked Vegetable Juice

Lunch: Berry Antioxidant Blend
Snack: Refreshing Hydration Mix
Dinner: Green Detox Juice

Day 3:
Breakfast: Berry Antioxidant Blend
Snack: Green Detox Juice
Lunch: Refreshing Hydration Mix
Snack: Citrus Immunity Booster
Dinner: ProteinPacked Vegetable Juice

Conclusion

Exploring resources such as recommended books and articles, joining online communities and support groups, and trying additional recipes and meal plans can enhance your juice cleanse experience. These resources provide valuable information, support, and inspiration to help you successfully navigate and maximize the benefits of your cleanse journey. Whether you're a beginner or seasoned cleanse enthusiast, leveraging these resources can contribute to a more informed and enjoyable cleanse experience while promoting overall health and wellbeing.